Elevate Your L… Guide to Health, Fitness, and Nutrition

Disclaimer:

The items within this book are not medical advice but suggestions on a better way to live your life. The information presented is based on personal experience, research, and professional insights but is not intended to diagnose, treat, cure, or prevent any condition.

Always consult with a qualified healthcare provider, physician, or registered dietitian before making any significant changes to your health, diet, exercise routine, or lifestyle—especially if you have underlying medical conditions or are taking medications.

The author and publisher disclaim any liability for injuries, losses, or damages incurred as a result of the use or misuse of the information provided herein.

Table of Contents

1. Introduction: The Journey to a Better You
2. The Mindset Shift: Your Foundation for Change
3. Nutrition Fundamentals: Fueling Your Body Right
4. Fitness for Every Body: Movement as Medicine
5. Holistic Wellness: More Than Just Diet and Exercise
6. Tracking Progress Without Obsession
7. Creating a Sustainable Routine
8. Navigating Setbacks: Progress is Not Linear
9. The Role of Vitamins & Supplements
10. Final Thoughts: Becoming Your Best Self
11. Resources and Further Reading
12. Self Reflection Through Journaling

Introduction: The Journey to a Better You

Welcome to *Elevate Your Life* — a guide crafted to help you take control of your health through practical, realistic, and sustainable actions. This book was designed for people who want to feel stronger, live better, and embrace a lifestyle that supports long-term wellness. We'll cover the essentials of fitness, nutrition, and mental well-being without overwhelming you or demanding perfection.

This is not a "one-size-fits-all" manual or a quick-fix fad. You will not find promises of instant abs or miracle diets. What you *will* find are tools, education, and encouragement rooted in real-world experience and research.

Whether you're starting from scratch, rebuilding after setbacks, or simply ready to level up, this guide is for you.

Let's begin your journey.

The Mindset Shift: Your Foundation for Change

Lasting transformation starts in the mind. Before you can improve your body, your habits, or your lifestyle, you must reshape how you think about health.

- **Redefine Success:** True success is consistency, not perfection. Small, repeatable actions compound over time.
- **Adopt a Growth Mindset:** Health is a journey, not a destination. Embrace learning and progress.
- **Ditch the All-or-Nothing Thinking:** Missing a workout or eating something indulgent doesn't mean failure. What matters is what you do next.

Shifting your mindset sets the tone for sustainable change. Believe you are capable—and that you are worth the effort.

Nutrition Fundamentals: Fueling Your Body Right

Nutrition is one of the most misunderstood and overwhelming aspects of health. But it doesn't have to be complicated. The goal is to create balance, not restriction.

- **Whole Foods First:** Focus on real, minimally processed foods—lean proteins, vegetables, fruits, whole grains, and healthy fats.
- **Hydration Matters:** Water supports digestion, energy levels, and cognitive function. Aim for at least 8 cups per day, more if you're active.
- **Understand Macronutrients:**
    - Protein builds and repairs tissues and supports metabolism.
    - Carbohydrates are your body's preferred source of energy.
    - Fats support hormone production and nutrient absorption.
- **Eat Mindfully:** Pay attention to hunger and fullness cues. Avoid multitasking while eating.
- **Balance Your Plate:** A good rule of thumb is to fill half your plate with vegetables, one-quarter with protein, and one-quarter with complex carbs.

Instead of chasing fad diets, **listen to your body, stay consistent, and make choices that align with how you want to feel. Nutrition is about nourishment, not punishment.**

Fitness for Every Body: Movement as Medicine

Fitness is not about achieving a certain body type — it's about honoring your body through movement. Regular physical activity improves energy levels, boosts mental health, and reduces the risk of chronic disease.

- **Start Where You Are:** You don't need to train like an athlete to reap the benefits of exercise. Walking, stretching, or bodyweight exercises are all excellent starting points.

- **Find Movement You Enjoy:** Whether it's dancing, swimming, hiking, or weightlifting, the best exercise is the one you'll stick to.

- **Mix It Up:** Include a combination of strength training, cardiovascular activity, flexibility work, and rest. This ensures well-rounded fitness and reduces injury risk.

- **Progress Over Perfection:** Track your effort, not just your results. Celebrate increased stamina, improved sleep, or a better mood.

Everybody is different. **Move in a way that respects your abilities while also challenging you to grow stronger.**

Holistic Wellness: More Than Just Diet and Exercise

True wellness integrates your mind, body, and spirit. It's about addressing the whole person and recognizing that health is more than what you eat or how you move.

- **Mental Health Matters:** Stress, anxiety, and burnout impact your physical health. Practices like journaling, meditation, and therapy can help you build emotional resilience.

- **Sleep is Non-Negotiable:** Quality sleep helps with hormone regulation, immune function, and recovery. Aim for 7–9 hours per night.

- **Environment and Relationships:** Your surroundings and social interactions affect your wellness. Cultivate supportive relationships and create a peaceful space.

- **Spiritual Practices:** Whether it's prayer, nature walks, mindfulness, or gratitude rituals, finding time to connect with something bigger than yourself can ground you.

A holistic approach helps you feel more balanced, empowered, and connected. Health is not just the absence of illness — it's a **state of thriving in every aspect of life**.

Tracking Progress Without Obsession

Tracking your journey is important—but only when done in a healthy, constructive way. It's easy to get caught up in numbers, photos, and comparisons, but real progress is so much more than that.

- **Measure What Matters:** Track energy levels, sleep quality, how your clothes fit, strength gains, or how you feel emotionally. The scale is just one data point.

- **Use Tools Wisely:** Journals, fitness apps, or progress photos can be helpful—but they should serve you, not control you.

- **Avoid Comparison Traps:** Everyone's path is unique. Celebrate *your* milestones, no matter how small.

- **Check In, Don't Obsess:** Set a rhythm for check-ins—weekly or monthly is usually enough. Don't let daily fluctuations drive your self-worth.

Progress is about becoming stronger, more aware, and more in tune with your body—not about chasing an ideal. Track your growth with **compassion, curiosity, and patience.**

Creating a Sustainable Routine

The goal isn't perfection—it's consistency. A sustainable routine is one that you can maintain long-term without burning out.

- **Start Small:** Begin with simple, manageable habits. One or two healthy choices daily are enough to gain momentum.
- **Schedule Your Wellness:** Treat your workouts, meal prep, and downtime like appointments. Block out time in your calendar.
- **Habit Stacking:** Tie a new habit to something you already do. For example, stretch after brushing your teeth or drink water before your morning coffee.
- **Adjust as You Go:** Life changes—your routine should too. Don't be afraid to modify your schedule when needed. Flexibility supports consistency.
- **Prioritize Recovery:** Rest is essential. Build in time for relaxation, sleep, and active recovery.

Consistency builds confidence. A routine that supports your lifestyle—not one that controls it—is the key to long-term success.

Navigating Setbacks: Progress is Not Linear

One of the most important truths about any health journey is this: progress is not a straight line. There will be ups and downs, and that's not just normal—it's expected.

- **Anticipate Obstacles:** Life will throw curveballs. Travel, stress, illness, or emotional upheavals can disrupt your routine. Having a flexible mindset prepares you to adapt instead of quit.

- **Reframe Setbacks as Lessons:** Instead of labeling a tough week as failure, ask: *What did I learn? What can I improve next time?*

- **Avoid the Guilt Spiral:** Skipping a workout or overindulging doesn't erase your progress. Let go of guilt and refocus with compassion.

- **Come Back with One Small Win:** When motivation is low, start with a small, achievable action—like drinking water or stretching. One step leads to the next.

- **Track Emotional Progress:** Sometimes, the biggest growth is invisible. Are you handling stress better? Setting boundaries? Feeling more self-aware?

Remember: real transformation is rarely linear. **Trust the process, give yourself grace, and stay the course.**

The Role of Vitamins & Supplements

Vitamins and supplements can play a supportive role in a well-rounded wellness routine, especially when dietary gaps or specific needs arise. However, not all supplements are created equal, and more isn't always better.

Why Supplements May Be Needed

- Nutrient Gaps: Even a well-balanced diet can fall short in key nutrients like Vitamin D, B12, or Iron.
- Life Stage Needs: Nutritional needs differ between genders and change with age, pregnancy, menopause, or athletic activity.
- Food Accessibility: Those in food deserts or with dietary restrictions may rely more on supplementation.
- Absorption Issues: Some medical conditions affect how well your body absorbs nutrients from food.

Gender-Specific Considerations

For Women:

- Iron: Especially important for menstruating women.
- Calcium & Vitamin D: Supports bone health, particularly during menopause.
- Folate: Essential during reproductive years for pregnancy planning.

For Men:

- Magnesium: Supports muscle recovery and heart health.
- Zinc: Important for immune function and testosterone balance.
- B Vitamins: Support energy levels and brain function.

Always tailor your supplement stack to your personal needs, lifestyle, and bloodwork when possible.

Importance of Third-Party Testing

Many supplements are unregulated, meaning what's on the label may not reflect what's in the bottle. Look for products certified by:

- NSF Certified for Sport
- USP (U.S. Pharmacopeia)
- Informed-Choice

These labels ensure the product has been tested for purity, potency, and safety, and is free from harmful contaminants or banned substances.

How to Use Supplements Safely

- Start with Food First: Supplements are *supplements*, not replacements.
- Avoid Overdosing: Fat-soluble vitamins like A, D, E, and K can accumulate and cause toxicity.
- Consult a Professional: Ideally, speak with a dietitian or physician before starting a new supplement, especially if you’re taking medication.

- Track Effects: Like any lifestyle change, observe how your body responds to supplementation and adjust accordingly.

When used wisely, **supplements can be a great tool to support your wellness journey**—but they should never replace a nutritious diet or a balanced lifestyle.

Final Thoughts: Becoming Your Best Self

By reaching this point in the guide, you've already taken a significant step toward becoming the healthiest, most empowered version of yourself. Remember, this journey isn't about quick fixes or chasing perfection—it's about growth, self-respect, and long-term vitality.

Here are the core truths to carry forward:

- ***Your Health is a Lifelong Investment***: The small choices you make each day matter. Every workout, every healthy meal, every act of self-care compounds over time.

- ***You Are Not Alone***: Communities, coaches, friends, and even books like this exist to support and uplift you. Lean on them.

- ***Flexibility is Strength***: Rigidity leads to burnout. Adaptability is what makes health sustainable.

- ***Progress is Personal***: Measure your growth by how you feel, how you show up in your life, and how you care for yourself—not by someone else's standards.

- ***Celebrate Your Wins***: Acknowledge your discipline, your consistency, and the fact that you're showing up for yourself.

Above all, stay committed to *yourself*. You are worthy of the time, energy, and attention that this journey requires. You don't have to be perfect—you just have to keep moving forward.

Let your transformation be about more than your body. Let it be about reclaiming your confidence, your peace, and your power.

Here's to elevating your life—one step at a time.

Resources and Further Reading

To help you continue your journey, here are trusted resources, tools, and communities that align with the holistic, evidence-based approach this guide promotes.

Nutrition and Wellness

- Precision Nutrition – www.precisionnutrition.com
- Harvard School of Public Health: Nutrition Source – www.hsph.harvard.edu/nutritionsource
- Cronometer (nutrition tracking app) – www.cronometer.com

Fitness & Exercise

- NASM (National Academy of Sports Medicine) – www.nasm.org
- Bodybuilding.com Exercise Database – www.bodybuilding.com/exercises
- Darebee (free at-home workouts) – www.darebee.com

Mindfulness & Mental Health

- Headspace (meditation app) – www.headspace.com
- The Science of Well-Being (Yale free course) – www.coursera.org/learn/the-science-of-well-being
- Therapy Directory (Psychology Today) – www.psychologytoday.com

Supplements and Safety

- Examine.com (evidence-based supplement database) – www.examine.com
- ConsumerLab (independent testing) – www.consumerlab.com
- USP Verified Supplements List – www.quality-supplements.org

Tracking Tools

- MyFitnessPal – for calorie and macro tracking
- Fitbit / Garmin / Apple Health – for activity and sleep monitoring
- Habitica – gamified habit tracking

Self Reflection Through Journaling

Self-reflective journaling is more than just putting pen to paper—it's a powerful tool for personal growth and transformation. By regularly exploring your thoughts, feelings, and experiences, you create a dedicated space to gain clarity, process emotions, and reinforce your goals. This practice helps you identify patterns, celebrate progress, and recognize areas for improvement without judgment.

In your health and wellness journey, journaling acts as a mirror, allowing you to track not only physical changes but also shifts in mindset and motivation. It encourages mindfulness and deepens self-awareness, making it easier to overcome setbacks and maintain long-term commitment.

Whether you're writing about your daily habits, challenges, or victories, self-reflective journaling fosters a compassionate and honest relationship with yourself—one that is essential for lasting change and holistic well-being.

Use these prompts on the next few pages to reflect, refocus, and elevate your mental wellness as you work through your health journey.

What does "healthy" mean to me right now?

Guided Reflection:

Health isn't a one-size-fits-all concept. Reflect on how your definition of health may have changed over time. What does being healthy look like for you mentally, physically, and emotionally? Think about what truly supports your well-being—not just what others say it should be.

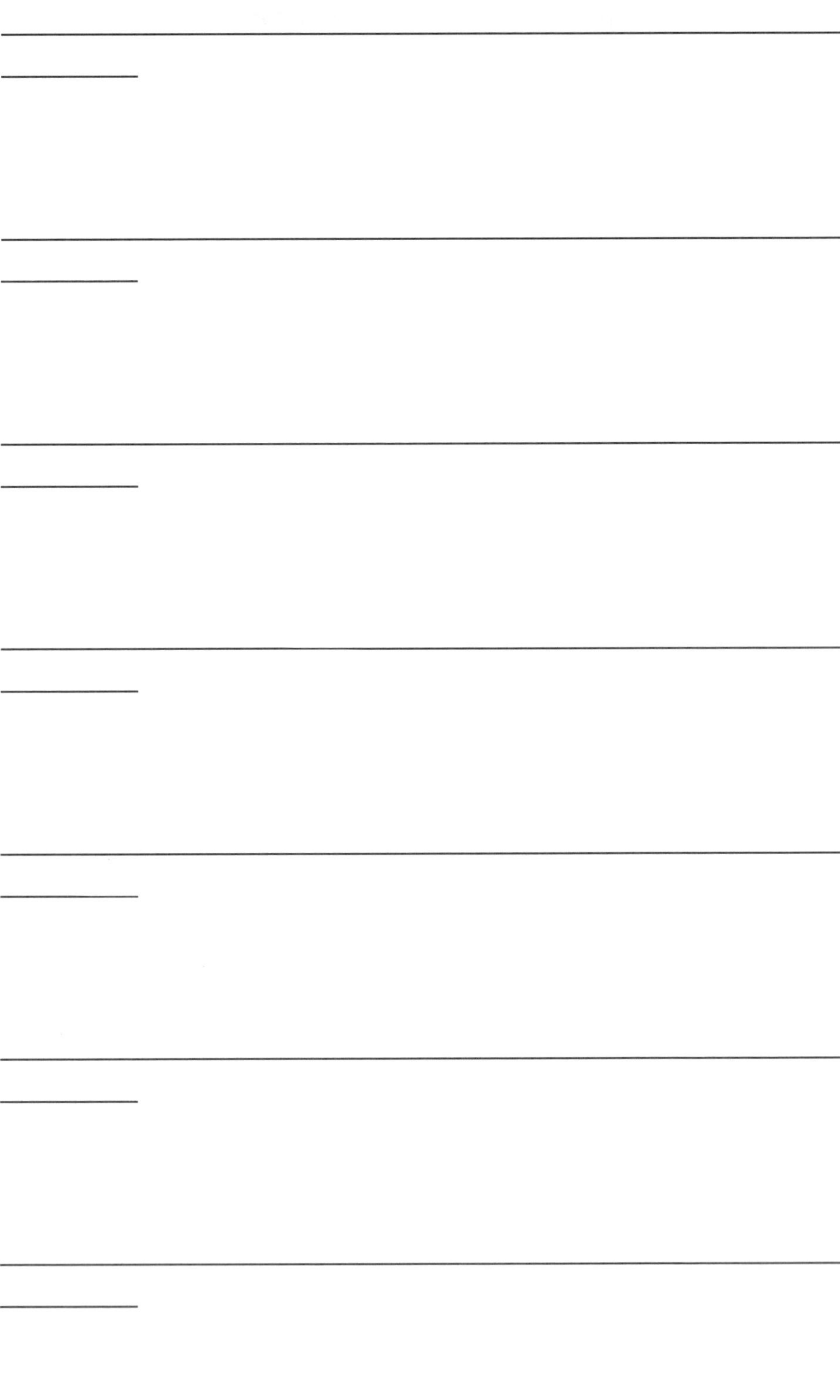

What's one habit I'm proud of developing lately?

Guided Reflection:

Pause and celebrate your growth. Think about a small or big habit you've built recently—whether it's drinking more water, setting boundaries, or moving your body. Why does this habit matter to you? What helped you stick with it, and how can you build on that momentum?

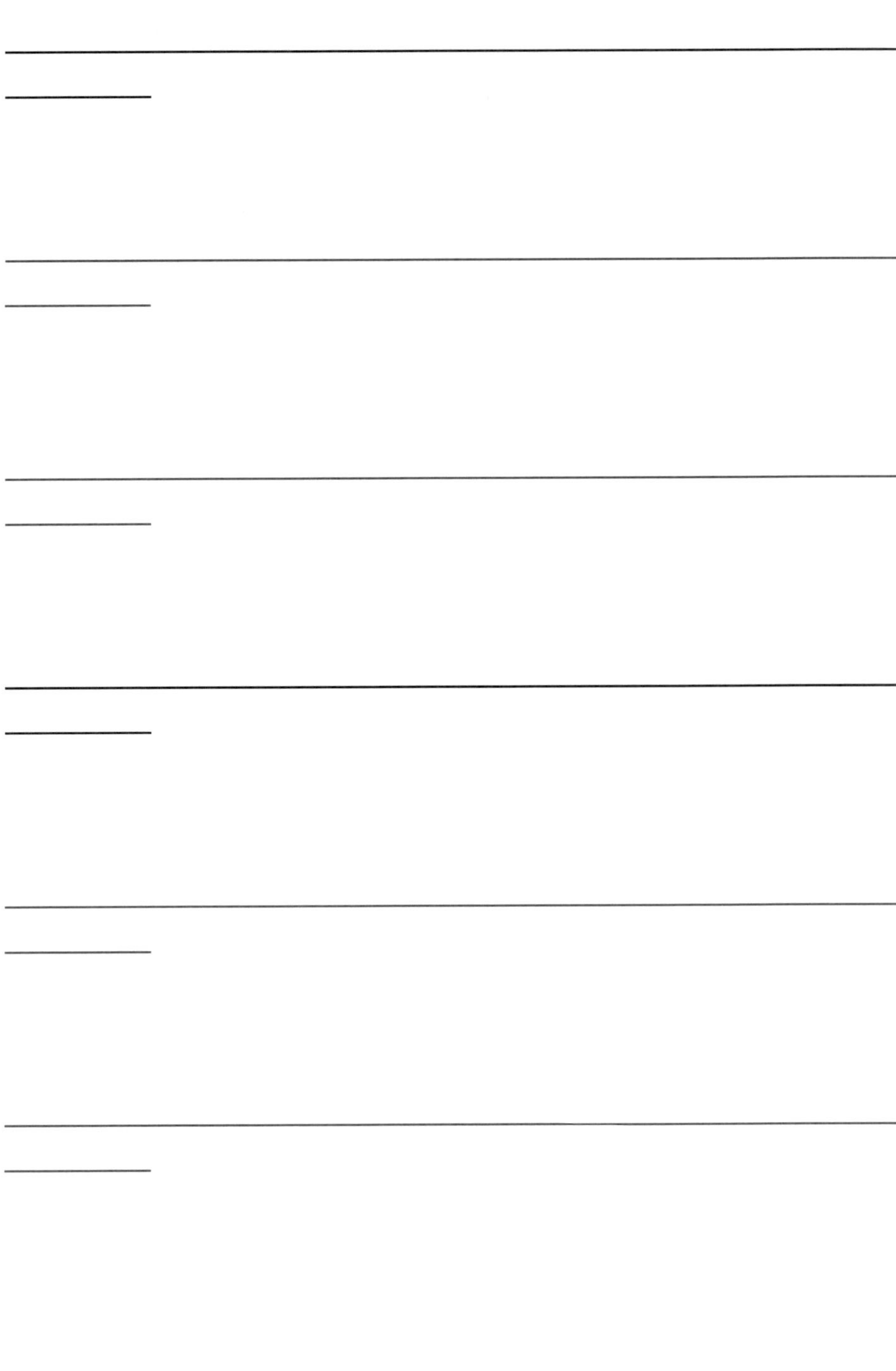

What's one limiting belief I need to let go of?

Guided Reflection:

We all carry thoughts that hold us back. Identify a belief you've internalized that no longer serves your goals or values. Where did it come from? What evidence challenges it? And what empowering belief could you replace it with?

When do I feel most confident and why?

Guided Reflection:

Think about the moments when you feel fully like yourself—energized, empowered, and aligned. What are you doing? Who are you with? These clues can help guide your choices and habits toward the things that nourish your spirit.

What's one area of my wellness that I'd like to improve this month?

Guided Reflection:

Wellness is multi-dimensional—physical, mental, emotional, spiritual. Take a moment to assess where you're feeling out of balance. Maybe it's your sleep, nutrition, movement, stress management, or social connection. Choose one area to gently focus on and set a small, achievable goal. What would support you best this month?

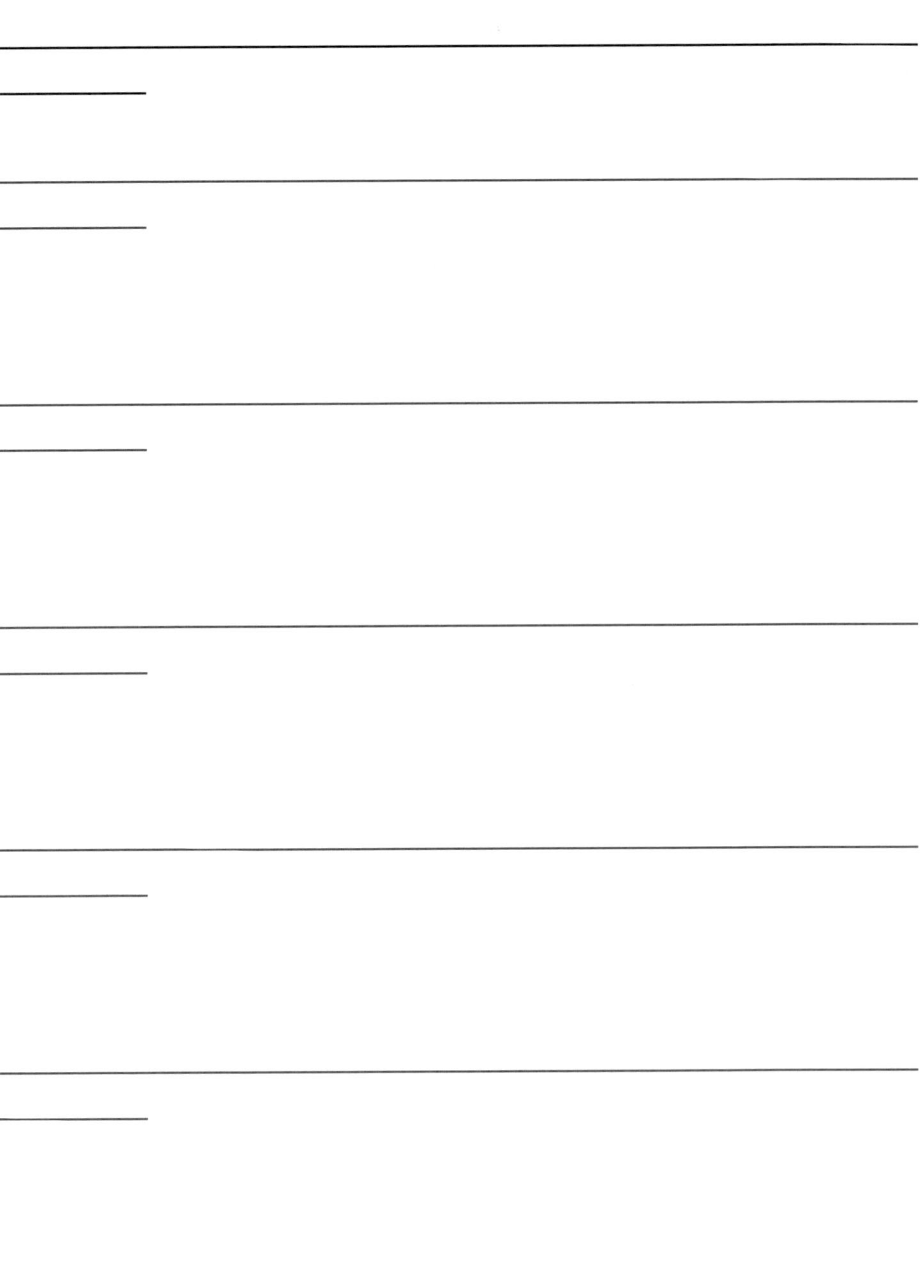

How do I talk to myself on bad days—and how can I do better?

Guided Reflection:

Our inner voice matters most when we’re struggling. Reflect on the language and tone you use with yourself during tough moments. Are you compassionate or critical? Encouraging or dismissive? Consider how you'd speak to a loved one—and explore how you can begin showing yourself the same grace.

About the Author

Hi! I'm Christian Gaskins—a certified Nutrition Care Specialist through the U.S. military, a former Division II collegiate athlete, and a lifelong fitness enthusiast who believes that health isn't just about how you look, but how you live.

My journey has taken me from competitive sports to military service, where I learned how discipline, mindset, and practical nutrition could work together to create lasting change. But more importantly, I learned that health doesn't need to be extreme—it needs to be sustainable, personal, and built for real life.

This book was created to share those lessons. Whether you're just starting out or trying to take your wellness to the next level, I wanted to offer something honest, encouraging, and actionable—because I've been where you are, and I know what works when life gets busy or motivation runs low.

When I'm not training, or building new ways to simplify healthy living, you'll find me lifting in the gym, spending time outdoors, playing the game with friends or trying to turn every meal into a macro-friendly masterpiece.

Let's stay connected and keep this journey going together.

Christian T Gaskins
📱 Instagram: GeeQFitness

Made in the USA
Columbia, SC
16 July 2025